WHO

HAS

YOUR

BACK

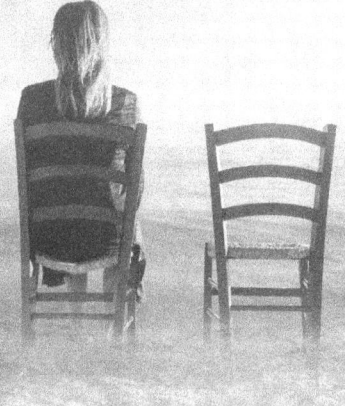

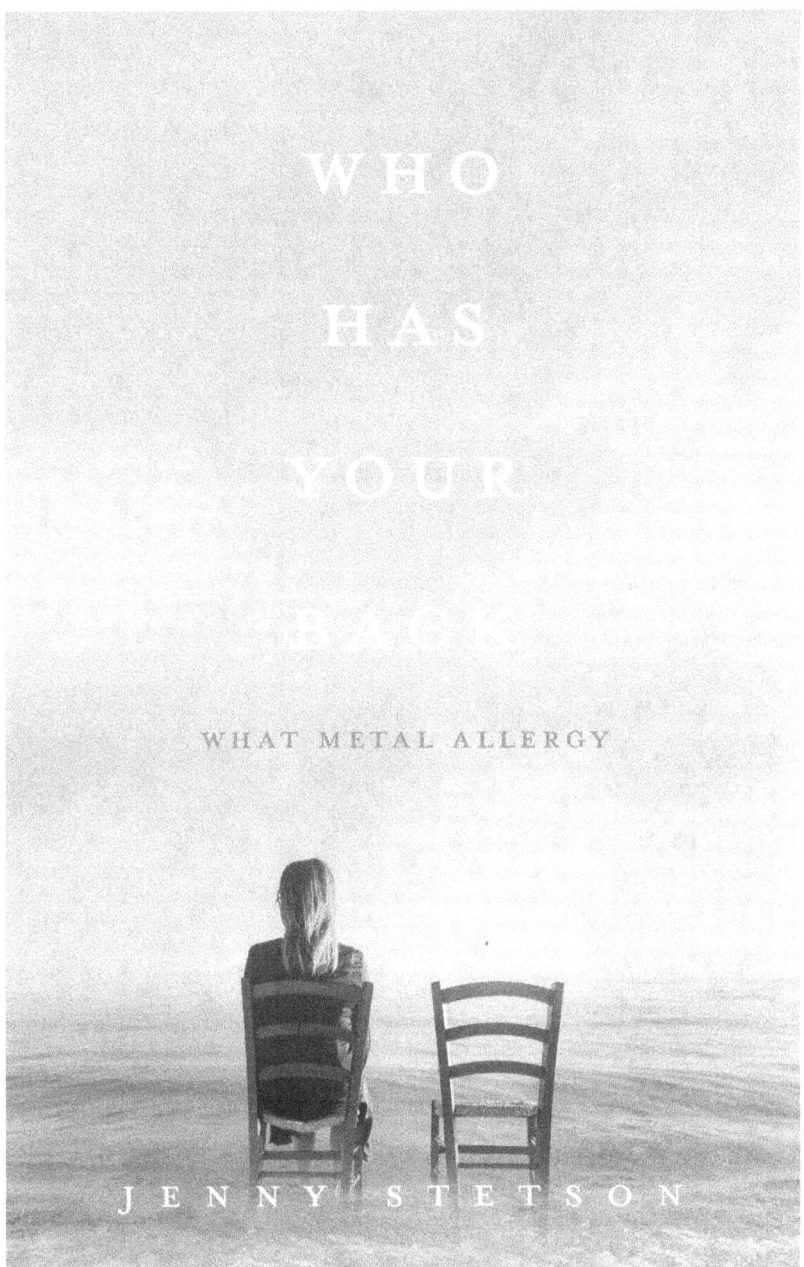

Xulon Press
2301 Lucien Way #415
Maitland, FL 32751
407.339.4217
www.xulonpress.com

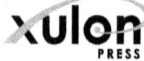

© 2023 by Jenny Stetson

All rights reserved solely by the author. The author guarantees all contents are original and do not infringe upon the legal rights of any other person or work. No part of this book may be reproduced in any form without the permission of the author.

Due to the changing nature of the Internet, if there are any web addresses, links, or URLs included in this manuscript, these may have been altered and may no longer be accessible. The views and opinions shared in this book belong solely to the author and do not necessarily reflect those of the publisher. The publisher therefore disclaims responsibility for the views or opinions expressed within the work.

Paperback ISBN-13: 978-1-66288-108-4
Ebook ISBN-13: 978-1-66288-109-1

INTRODUCTION

My name is Jenny Stetson. I am a fifty-six-year-old female, and I was born and raised in Santa Maria, California. I was born with many allergies: allergies to foods, lotions, plants, grass, trees, juices, etc. As a result of this, I suffered from asthma and tonsillitis, and was often sick with breathing difficulties, fevers, or rashes.

As a small child, after playing outside, my parents had often taken me to the doctor's office for adrenaline shots or breathing treatments. At least twice a year, when I came down with tonsillitis, my fevers had gone upward to 104° or 105° and I was packed in ice. My vision was affected from the high temperatures, and eventually, I was prescribed glasses in order to see at a young age. My vision then was 20/200.

As I grew up, my body adapted to these allergies. I kind of outgrew the symptoms. However, seasonal asthma seems to remain, even today. Treatment for asthma required over-the-counter allergy medications, a prescribed albuterol inhaler, or nebulizer. I had discovered that I was allergic to certain metals as well, after I had my ears pierced when I was ten. Certain metals in jewelry broke me out in a rash or made me itch. I was also extremely allergic to primula and poison oak.

Growing up, I was somewhat of a tomboy. I enjoyed the outdoors, climbing trees, skating, and riding bikes. In high school, I loved track, swimming, and gymnastics. I hung out with a water polo team, cheerleaders, and was also on the drill team. I was athletic and active.

My all-time dream job was law enforcement. Although I had worked many jobs, none of them were permanent careers. I had two college degrees, and in my thirties, I followed that dream and went into law enforcement. At that time, I was a single, divorced woman with two kids. I worked full-time at my job and attended the police academy during nights and weekends. After graduating the academy, I was hired with the city of Guadalupe, California, in 1996. I worked with the city of Guadalupe for four-and-a-half years. I was laterally hired by the Santa Barbara County Sheriff's Department in 2000. In the year 2010, my law enforcement career was cut short, since I had gone out on a shoulder and back injury, and eventually retired disabled in 2016.

Most of my life I had been healthy, meaning that I was rarely sick other than allergies. I took good care of my body, stayed in shape, and ate well. I rarely consumed alcohol and didn't smoke or use recreational drugs. I never got tattoos. I've never broken any bones ; however, I was involved in many automobile collisions, most of which were not my fault. I only suffered bruises and scrapes from the accidents.

Currently, I am a retired, disabled Santa Barbara County Deputy Sheriff Coroner. I am writing and sharing my story, in the hope of educating others. At the time that I had gone through this in 2009, many of the California doctors in the Santa Maria, Arroyo Grande,

Santa Barbara County area, as well as the Los Angeles area, were unaware of metal allergies. The mindset among care was that the side effect or reaction from the synthetic implant was rare. Because of this, doctors didn't share this with their patients, or even consider it was a reason for the failed surgery. It was kind of shoved aside and ignored.

Having gone through this, I can say that I experienced this firsthand, and many of the doctors I spoke with denied that it was a reason for my rashes, bleeding, headaches, and lymphedema. I literally found out the hard way. Everything I am writing today is firsthand experience that I personally went through, and is not intended to point fingers at anyone or slander any doctors. The intent of this book is to educate those undergoing an orthopedic implant surgery. Each patient should do their own research prior to jumping into it. If you have any pre-existing conditions or allergies, it would behoove you to look further into the components of any orthopedic implant, and possibly have blood allergy tests conducted prior to any surgery.

I would hate to see anybody else go through what I suffered through after undergoing the surgery. It was nothing short of horrific. Additionally, and I hate to admit it, but I first-hand experienced it: medical doctors treat females different than males. For instance, instead of looking at the scientific reason for any of the symptoms I had, I was sent to an OBGYN for hormone treatments, a psychologist, and even a psychiatrist. Quite often, I was prescribed medication for depression, pain, or other symptoms that I had. None of the medical doctors looked into the reason for my reactions; they simply reacted to the side-effect symptoms.

Had I not been an advocate for myself, I can most certainly say my outcome would have been more detrimental, or even fatal. Everyone believed the doctors because they are *doctors*. I mean how could that many doctors be wrong? So, I continue with this story in the hopes that this will reach the right people, and hopefully help somebody else avoid suffering like I did.

A lot of people whom I worked with, as well as friends of mine, were not aware of how dangerous my situation was with the metal allergy. Had I not been an advocate and fought, I most likely wouldn't be here today telling my story. I would be dead.

THE JOURNEY

My journey began in the year 2009. At that time, I was employed with the County of Santa Barbara Sheriff Department as the Deputy Sheriff/Coroner on patrol. I began my career with this agency in the year 2000 and worked until December of 2010. This was the year that I went out on a back injury. I wasn't physically retired until 2016, since this was a work comp-related injury, and was dragged out. Nothing happens overnight when a claim is filed, and it turns into a huge claim like mine. Once a claim is filed, authorization is needed for referrals to see doctors, or to have tests conducted, and sometimes, several months would pass while I waited for these authorizations.

On top of that, dealing with attorneys is another issue. Several days and/or weeks had passed between each appointment. Being prescribed ineffective medication and fighting for some relief from one doctor to another, while awaiting authorization, seemed like a lifetime when one is in horrific pain and suffering. In addition, one Workers' Compensation doctor often referred me to another doctor as a result of my symptoms, and authorization had to be made prior to a visit. Often, this took several weeks or months. I had to make many phone calls to the adjuster to get things expedited.

Looking back, I recall that my symptoms began with restless leg cramping, and tingling in my hips down both legs. I had some lower back pain. The aching in my legs required me to pull over, get out, and walk around for a bit. At that time, I wasn't sure if it was due to sitting too much. The weight of the gun belt and the position of the belt often caused issues while sitting in a patrol car. This was because of all the equipment on the gun belt, which pushed into the back and hips while sitting and driving. Over time, I noticed that the symptoms seemed to worsen rather than go away, no matter what I did. I tried over-the-counter muscle relaxers, such as Aleve or Tylenol. I went in for massages three to four times a week. Everything I had done provided some relief, but it wasn't a permanent solution, and the symptoms kept coming back and aggravating me.

Following the cramping and tingling, I noticed that I had lower back pain and weakness. I wasn't able to lift my duty bag out of the trunk, which required me to slightly bend over, reach in, and lift the bag out. The duty bag probably weighed thirty to forty pounds, and contained issued property required to keep with me at all times. I also had a second duty bag, which contained legal documents, penal and vehicle code books, citations, and miscellaneous property needed for my job, which I kept strapped in the front seat on the passenger side. It weighed about thirty to forty pounds. I also wore a bulletproof vest and black military-type boots.

After a month or so had passed, the aggravating symptoms worsened. I noticed it had become difficult to get out of the driver's seat, due to my back stiffening and locking. I couldn't swivel my legs to the side in order to exit. I had also experienced a loss of bowel and bladder control, and a few times, I barely made it to the restroom.

The pain was so horrific that I couldn't tell if I had to go, or didn't have to go, which delayed me getting there in time to relieve myself.

I reported my symptoms to my supervisor and began a Workers' Compensation claim. I was referred to a Work Comp clinic, where x-rays were taken and I was examined. I filled out several forms explaining how I had gotten injured, and the symptoms that I had. The forms were given to the doctor to review. The Work Comp clinic MD circled "female problems" on the paperwork, and stated my complaints were not validated. The MD told me that my reported pain had nothing to do with work. I questioned the MD and asked him why he circled "female problems," when I clearly had gone in there with a back injury complaint. I was vocal about my situation, and the MD turned and ignored me.

I made an appointment with my primary care physician regarding my back pain. My primary care physician requested an x-ray and an MRI of my spine. My family care doctor was aware that I had a partial hysterectomy when I was twenty-one, and the final hysterectomy in 2008. I no longer had menstrual cycles, nor was I taking any hormone therapy. I rarely had gotten sick, and all my bloodwork and physical exams were up to date, stating I was healthy. My family care doctor also told me that the MRI reported a tear in the L5 lumbar, and wrote a note for my employer, relieving me from work for a few days. While at home, I iced my lower back, and did light stretches and walking as prescribed. I invested in a lumbar brace to wear during the daytime for support. If I could describe the amount of pain I suffered, it would be like cutting both my legs off without any pain medication. I lost both bowel and bladder control, and was in such aggravating pain, I wasn't sure if I had to go to the bathroom or not . I felt as if my bladder was full but it wasn't. By the time I got to the bathroom, it was too late. Sometimes, I cried in my sleep, not even knowing it. My spouse had even asked me to go into the other room, so he could sleep. Several months had passed with me in this horrific pain. I had made several trips to the emergency room for pain control, which became a burden on my family. I felt like a burden to everyone. I couldn't return back to work in this pain, and the doctors didn't seem to believe me, or were ignoring me treatment. I became depressed as a result. I had annoying pain, and I had no way to control it. I went to a dark place in my life, and considered ending it. I prayed many nights for help and guidance with what I was going through.

I tried many ways to escape from the pain: meditating, sewing, and reading books. I spent hours outside on a swing, meditating with the sounds of nature. Sometimes, I would go out in the backyard and do light gardening. The peaceful outdoors, with birds chirping and the sun on my body, were soothing and a great distraction. Even after medicating, I had difficulty keeping the pain from driving me crazy. At one point, I had so much pain that I was clenching my jaw in my sleep without realizing it. This caused jaw and headache pain. After a year and a half of doing this, I eventually cracked a molar. I sought help with my dentist and explained that I thought I cracked a molar. He told me I seemed relaxed about the ordeal, and told me that I would be in a lot of pain if I had cracked a molar. I told him I *was* in a lot of pain. The dentist said I appeared quite calm for someone who cracked a molar. Trying to keep my sense of humor, I asked the dentist, "If I threw myself on the floor and started crying, would I get treatment?"

The dentist laughed, sat me in the chair, and examined my right rear molar. Sure enough, it was cracked. The dentist told me that I must handle pain very well. The dentist told me that patients with cracked molars typically came in crying and emotional. Anyway, he repaired my cracked molar, and I was sent on my way.

THE TREATMENT

After consulting with a Workers' Compensation attorney, I was referred to a neurosurgeon in Santa Barbara. The neurosurgeon ordered x-rays, as well as an MRI. The test results revealed a tear in my L5. From there, I was referred to physical therapy. I went through twenty-four visits of physical therapy, with no positive results. The therapy only seemed to aggravate my pain. I only saw this doctor maybe once or twice a month, so several weeks had passed between each visit. Trying to get answers seemed like forever, and there was no light at the end of my tunnel for relief.

The MD neurosurgeon recommended another test — Intrathecal MRI — which went up into the inside of the spine. I can't remember if he explained the possible side effects from this test at that time. I was willing to do about anything to find some relief or answers. The x-ray tech who conducted this test gave me a spinal tap. However, he was supposed to wait until my back was numb. He began the exam before my spine was numb, and went up inside with the camera. It was extremely painful and felt like a bottle brush going up into my spine. I was crying and in pain; the tech told me to remain calm and to please not move. Although the test was quick, it was extremely painful. I had urinated myself and had tears running down my cheeks from the ordeal. The test results revealed degenerative disc disease, two ruptured discs, and pinched nerves. Following this test, I was placed in a room to rest prior to being released.

A few hours after returning home from that test, my whole right leg went cold and numb. My whole leg down to my foot fell asleep. I could not feel my leg when I walked. I often tripped or slipped on the stairs in my house because I couldn't feel my leg on the stairs. My leg remained this way for several weeks. I had even gone in for a pedicure, where my feet were placed in a warm soak bath. The pedicurist, after removing my foot from the warm bath, appeared shocked, and told me my foot was cold. She had never experienced anybody having a cold foot coming out of a warm bath before. I laughed and told her that's my cold foot. The pedicurist seemed extremely concerned. I explained to her why it was that way.

Upon returning to the MD neurosurgeon, he and I decided that a synthetic disc implant would be the best option for me, as it had great patient outcomes, and patients were able to return to work full duty. The MD neurosurgeon showed me the device, which was made of metal, had two separate discs attached, and rotated for flexion in the spine, similar to a real spine disc. I noted the metal on the disc and asked the doctor if anybody had reported problems with the device or reactions. I questioned failed surgery. The doctor told me that he had implanted over 200 synthetic implants, the side effects were rare, and none of his patients had ever experienced anything like that. He convinced me that this was my best option, so I agreed to the surgery. Prior to the surgery being authorized by Workers' Comp, I was required to see two additional orthopedic doctors for a second and third opinion.

Several months later, Workers' Comp finally authorized the disc replacement surgery, which took place at a Santa Barbara hospital outpatient. Waking up from the surgery, I did feel better; however, my bladder had bothered me. I was kept overnight for observation. Before I was released, I mentioned to the nurse about my bladder feeling full, and how it bothered me. The RN told me I had emptied my bladder sufficiently enough, and that it probably was the result of back pain feeling like bladder pain. I was discharged and sent home. When I got home, I went to bed. I slept a few hours and woke up in severe pain, doubled over. My family rushed me to the emergency room for treatment. The emergency room medical doctor did immediate scans, gave me pain medication, and stated that my bladder was so full, that it almost ruptured. Additionally, I had a bowel blockage. They catheterized me to empty my bladder, and did an enema to flush my bowels. I was sent home with a referral to a gastroenterologist and a urologist for further treatment.

A few days had passed after the surgery and I was scheduled to see pain management regarding my post-op medications. My father drove me and there were so many people in the waiting room that I had to sit in my walker. The next thing I knew, I was on the floor, with a bunch of people standing around me. I had passed out and fallen face-first into the floor. My father had gone out to the car and was unaware that I had passed out as he had been outside. My father was promptly notified by the other patients that I had fallen. Apparently, I had passed out head-first into the carpet, and had a severe scrape on my eye. The doctor's office notified medics. The ambulance medics scooped me up and transported me to the hospital for treatment. My father told me that there were so many people in that small room, there wasn't enough seating or oxygen, so even he had to go outside for air. Some of the patients were waiting on the floor, as there were not enough chairs.

When I finally got my appointment with the MD gastroenterologist, we discussed my symptoms and he believed the medication possibly slowed my bowels, causing constipation. I was prescribed over-the-counter stool softeners, and a colonoscopy was scheduled. The over-the-counter stool softeners did not seem to help. I tried Miralax, Dulcolax Sodium, and Ex-lax, as well as the use of saline enemas. After taking the colonoscopy medication, which flushed me out, the results of the colonoscopy were normal, with no noted problems. At this point, the MD gastroenterologists believed my pain meds had possibly caused the bowels not to move.

Several months had passed, and I had several visits with this MD gastroenterologist. We tried numerous different medications, none of which seem to be a long-term solution. A year later, additional different symptoms were noted from taking some of these medications, and had caused further complications. A couple years later, I had internal bleeding and had passed large blood clots in my bowels, which were concerning to me.

The MD gastroenterologist ordered another colonoscopy, which was normal; however, there was notable bleeding. He was unable to determine where the blood was coming from, but did note that there was bleeding. Additionally, I had internal and external hemorrhoids, which was a direct result of the constipation. The MD neurologist suggested banding for the internal hemorrhoids, since they would cause medical complications with a bowel movement. Banding of hemorrhoids is where the doctor slips a tight rubber and around the hemorrhoid to cut off the blood supply and it dries out.

The external hemorrhoids were to be treated with over-the-counter medication, and soaking in a tub. The first time I had a hemorrhoid banding, I was walking out of the office and passed out. I grabbed the doctor's jacket, as I fell to the floor. The MD was terrified, as he had never seen a patient go through this. It was a side effect from the procedure; however, he had never seen it. A family member of mine was notified about my condition, and responded to take me to the emergency room. My blood pressure had dropped so low that the MD almost called a medic. Once I was in the emergency room, I was given pain medication, and my blood pressure went back up. The ER doctor stated that my back pain was so severe, that the banding put me in shock. Over the years following that appointment, I had to have two additional banding procedures. Because of what I experienced on the first one, I had to bring a driver with me.

I saw the MD urologist regarding my bladder not emptying. The MD urologist did several tests, and determined I had a neurogenic bladder, most likely as a result of the back surgery causing nerve damage. I was prescribed individual disposable self-catheters, and advised proper protocol for monitoring this type of condition. I continued seeing this MD urologist for over three years, with no improvements. I had gotten severe bladder infections from not emptying my bladder sufficiently, and also from the lymphedema issues. The toxicity from the lymphedema made my urine smelsl horrible.

Meanwhile, during all these other appointments I was attending, I had put on water weight, which started around my abdominal truncal area and spread into my arms, hands, and eventually down my body. I wasn't eating enough to gain weight and could not figure out why I was putting weight *on*. I mentioned this to the Workers' Comp doctors, and was told that it's ok to gain weight. I expressed my concern that I wasn't eating enough to gain weight and didn't feel well. I felt bloated and nauseated, with migraines on top of my other symptoms. Because of this, it made hydrating and eating difficult. None of the Work Comp doctors seemed concerned about my symptoms, and advised me to make an appointment with my primary care physician.

So, I made an appointment with my primary care physician, *again*, whom I had gone to for over twenty years. My family care doctor was concerned, since he had never seen me in this kind of condition. He had seen me just prior to my surgery. My family care doctor believed that everything I was going through was directly tied to the surgery somehow. My blood pressure was high; my pulse was high. I had gained eighty pounds and had rashes, bladder and bowel trouble, migraines, all of which I had never had before. I was agitated and emotional when I spoke to the family care doctor. We discussed the possibility that I had lymphedema, and I was referred to a therapist who treated lymphedema. I was prescribed anti-anxiety and migraine medication.

A few weeks later, I saw the lymphedema physical therapist. She noted that I had a severe case of lymphedema, and made three appointments a week for massages to reduce the fluid in my body. After a few weeks, she reduced the visits to twice a week. I had to invest in compression garments for my entire body. The compression nylons went up to my belly, and I had a torso abdominal garment that slid up and went to my chest. There was a chest garment that snapped in the front, and then one for each arm. Every morning, I had to put these on, and every night, I had to take them off and wash them. I saw this physical therapist for three years in order to control my lymphedema, which never seemed to go away. I had gained so much weight that my shoes didn't fit. I normally wore clothing size medium, a size seven to eight. Because of the lymphedema, I was in a size twelve. My belly was distended from the water weight. The lymphedema made me sweat and stink, and I could not wash the odor away. This was very embarrassing to me and depressed me severely. It was almost like being pregnant all over again. I was so bloated and nauseated that it was difficult to eat or drink. The migraines made me vomit daily, which gave me bloody noses and back pain. I had to take Zofran for nausea twice daily in order to drink and eat. Numerous visits were made to the emergency room in order to get rehydrated, and they gave me IV's with pain meds.

Another symptom I noticed was loss of hearing. I had experienced hearing difficulty as a result of the buzzing and ringing in both of my ears. I made an appointment with an MD ENT-Otolaryngologist. After conducting a hearing exam, the hearing doctor had determined that I was legally tone deaf. I explained to him that I was a deputy sheriff and had gotten injured on the job, had undergone a lumbar disc replacement surgery, and had a reaction from the implant. The doctor excused himself and returned with a printed piece of paper, which he had found online. The article talked about chromium cobalt and metal allergies causing hearing losses, which were irreversible and permanent. The MD explained that hearing aids would not work either because of the type of hearing loss it was.

The Santa Barbara County Workers' Compensation referred me to a psychiatrist and psychologist for mental health treatments, as I was displaying PTSD and depression symptoms related to the medication and pain symptoms that I was going through. They determined I was severely damaged at this point, but not dangerous. Although depressed and anxious, I was not a threat to myself or anybody else.

I continued seeing all these doctors, and eventually was referred to a neurologist to monitor the medication for nerve damage. The neurologist saw me for a period of two years, until he retired. There were no other neurologists in the area, and the orthopedic doctors were given the task of monitoring the nerve damage medication.

Workers' Compensation assigned me to a pain management MD, who was responsible for monitoring all my pain meds. I saw the same pain management doctor throughout these three years. After the first year, a spine stimulator was implanted in my left hip. The first implant was a non-chargeable battery, with wires going up my spine. My body drained the battery within the first few weeks, so I had to have a second spinal stimulator implanted. They removed the battery and replaced it with a rechargeable battery, which I still have today. I was also treated with cervical and spinal injections to control the pain and swelling in my spine. I also was given injections for my migraines.

I had never felt so alone in my entire life going through all of this. Many of the doctors had never dealt with anything like this, so they either referred me to another doctor, a psychologist, or told me everything was fine. Everything *wasn't* fine. I didn't have the best support system under my roof at home either. It was, quite frankly, the most horrific time of my life. I lived in constant pain, was severely depressed, bloated, and couldn't go to the bathroom, had migraines, and still had a family at home to take care of. I became a burden to my family, going doctor-to-doctor, and with emergency room visits. All of this I was going through was affecting my marriage severely, which added to my problems. That's a whole other ball of wax right there.

The shoulder injury I had in 2007, which was a shotgun recoil causing a torn rotator cuff and frozen shoulder, had never really healed. During all the lumbar and cervical issues with lymphedema, my shoulder was giving me trouble as well. Carpal tunnel had formed in my right arm, affecting my hand and wrist. There was nothing I could do until I took care of my lumbar and cervical issues first.

Two years had now passed by with the same symptoms, only now I was passing blood clots with my bowels. I had been researching all over the internet online in an attempt to find some sort of answers or solutions to everything I was going through. I ended up contacting the company that manufactured the synthetic disk which was in my spine. I telephoned them and spoke to several employees, and was advised that I possibly had an allergic reaction to the components of the disk. The company advised me they did not staff an allergist, but they did have a lab that they worked directly with. They referred me to this blood allergy lab in Chicago and advised me to let my doctor and attorneys know.

I looked up this lab and made telephone contact with them. I was mailed the blood allergy kit. Once I received the kit, a few days later, I took it to a phlebotomist, where the blood was drawn. I mailed the kit back to the ortho lab. I received the results via e-mail, which showed I was allergic to titanium and some other metals.

During this whole process, I had gotten two of these orthopedic blood allergy tests. The first blood allergy test was drawn when the synthetic device was still inside my spine. Two years later, the second blood allergy test was conducted after the synthetic disc had been removed, and prior to implanting a spine stimulator. My pain management MD requested the test, since he was authorized to implant a spine stimulator and didn't know if I would have a reaction to the components. Oddly, the test results were completely different. Once the implant was removed, the blood allergy test result showed that I was off the charts allergic to chromium cobalt and nickel.

I was referred to Cedar Sinai Spine Center for a second opinion, and began treatment with them. The doctors at Cedars Sinai had done everything they could to not cut into me, and now concluded that removal of the disc was absolutely necessary in order to save my life. At this point, my health was deteriorating. I was scheduled for in-patient surgery, which was approximately three hours long. The danger involved with the removal of a disc from my spine was explained to me, and they told me it was a life-threatening surgery. I was advised that I had a sixty-five percent chance of not surviving this surgery, and had to sign a death waiver. The doctor was sympathetic, and also explained that eventually, I would have toxic shock if the disc was not removed from my spine. I had a better chance on the operating table than not taking it. Although I was brave and agreed to the surgery; honestly, I was scared to death and put my faith in God. I trusted this surgeon with all my heart and knew that if anyone could help me, he could.

THE RECOVERY

The night before my surgery was a rough night. I wrote a letter to my family in the event that I did not survive the surgery, which entailed life insurance and wishes for my children and spouse. I spent the day outdoors with animals, crying and talking to Jesus. That night when I went to bed, I had a vivid dream, but I'm almost certain it was real. I was walking through the garden, and there was a beautiful archangel calling my name. He summoned me over and told me he needed to talk to me about what I was about to go through. He told me not to be afraid, and that I was strong, and he put his hand on my shoulder. When his hand touched my shoulder, all the pain in my body dissipated. It was the most amazing thing. He told me he was Gabriel, and he would be with me through the entire surgery, and not to fear because everything would be okay. Gabriel told me it would be a rough haul, and that I was going to go through a lot, but in the end, everything was going to get better.

During the removal of the disc surgery, the MD spine surgeon went in through the abdominal front but was not able to get to the disc. My body was turned over and an attempt was made through the back. The surgeons had the same problem, and were unable to remove the disc, since it had corroded in my spine. Additional surgeons were called in to assist. I had six surgeons, with additional assistants, now attempting to remove the disc and save my life. Eventually, they decided to cut my body in half from the belly button to the right hip muscle in order to bend the body and chisel the device out. Once they had made contact with the synthetic device, they realized it had corroded in my spine and there was no longer metal on it. It just looked like pieces of rocks in my spine. I was told they had to chisel the disc from my spine with a hammer and a straight tool. The disc was replaced with cadaver bone, a cage, plates, and screws. The totality of the surgery took eight-and-a-half hours, with blood transfusions, and ten days in the ICU. I awoke with IV's in my neck, ankles, and arms. From that point forward, I steadily improved each day that I was in there. I finally started to recover and heal.

I recall being saturated in sweat, as my body flushed the lymphedema and toxins from my body. The nurses had to remove the saturated, sweaty sheets, and sponge bathe my body. After a few days, I was able to get up and walk around, shower, and do physical therapy. By the time I was discharged, I had shrunk from a size ten to a size one, and my underwear didn't fit. My body, by sweating, flushed out the lymphedema toxins from my body, and reduced the swelling. I felt so much better, but was at bed rest for some time due to the incisions in the front, back, and the side of my torso. Once up and about on foot, however, I felt so much better that I hardly noticed the pain from the incisions. My right hip had the most pain. It felt like a rod with screws had been surgically implanted, which restricted my movements and sitting.

Following this surgery, several of the medications I had been taking were removed by the MD spine surgeon since they were no longer necessary. I saw this MD spine surgeon for approximately a year post-op, and was eventually discharged. When I was admitted, I was on nine different medications for different problems. All but three of these medications were no longer necessary to take. The surgery was a complete success, but not without side effects, as a result of the surgical incisions necessary to save my life.

My doctor referred me to psychiatric care following the surgery since I displayed symptoms of PTSD from stress, loud noises, or quick movements. Every now and then, I still had migraines and/or spinal headaches, but over time, they seemed to lessen. On one incident, we had stopped to eat lunch after an appointment. While eating in the cafeteria, someone dropped a plate, which broke, and the noise caused me to shake and turn three shades of white. I was advised that the symptoms I had were a direct result of my body fighting for its life from the toxic metals and surgeries I had to undergo to remove them. Although I have slowly improved over the years, I do notice that stress doesn't roll off my back as easily as it did prior to any of this horror story.

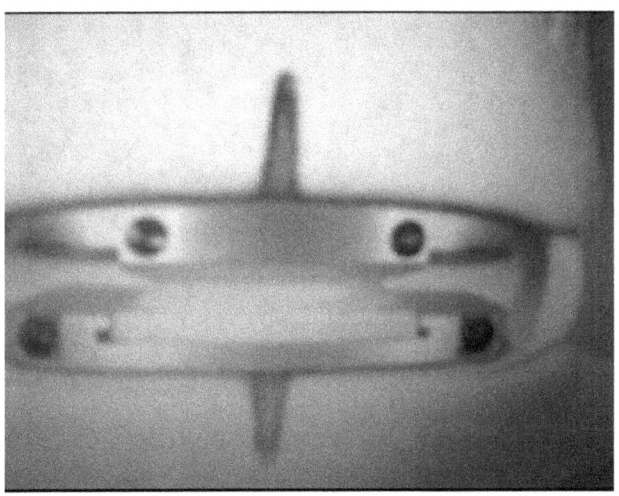

Here is a picture of the synthetic disc prior to surgery:

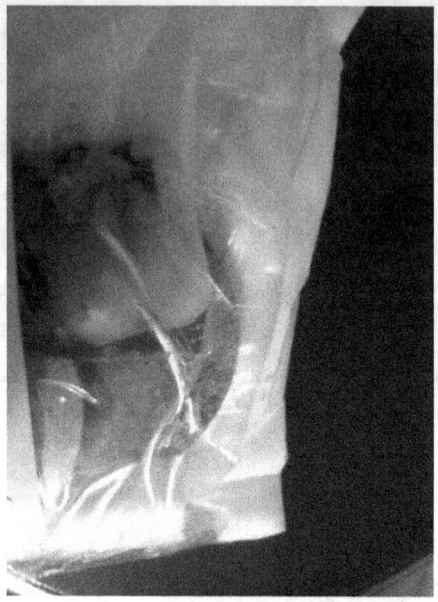

Here is a picture of the discs after being removed from my spine:

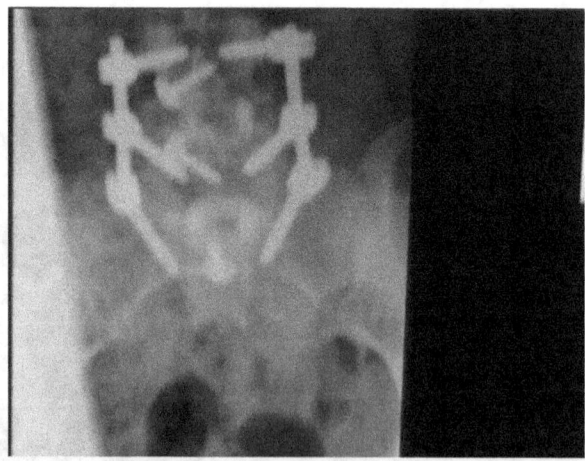

Here are x-rays of my post-operative spine after removing the synthetic disc and implanting cadaver bone, café, plates, and screws.

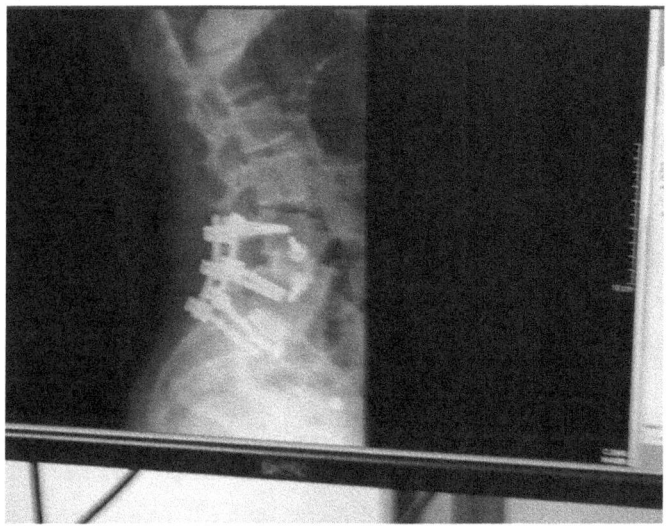

A year post-op, I was referred to a local orthopedic surgeon for pain management treatment, and continued orthopedic follow-up treatment. This entailed spinal injections, a spine stimulator surgically installed in my left hip, and partial removal of plates and screws that were no longer necessary once my back was fused. Although I had improved immensely, I had trouble sitting, standing, or walking long distances. At that time, I was only able to walk approximately ten minutes before dragging my leg and having to sit down. I continued getting neuropathy down my right leg and into my right foot, which caused neuromas on the bottom of my foot pad. I sought care at a podiatrist, who did injections via the top, and eventually had to surgically remove the neuroma through the top.

It still came back. I saw a surgical MD podiatrist at Cedar Sinai, who was able to remove the neuroma via the bottom pad of my foot beneath my second and fourth toes. My foot began to heal after this; however, there was still a small hole in the bottom of my foot. Every now and then when walking, it gives me grief, but so far the neuroma has not returned. I still have pain in the right foot similar to when a foot falls asleep, and it also feels swollen. The surgical MD stated that the neuroma was a definite reaction from my back surgery, and all the complications that went with it. Once my foot was able to heal, I was able to slowly start doing walks around the neighborhood to get my agility back up and strengthen my legs and back. To this day, it's difficult to sit too long or sit in certain positions.

If I sit too long in a chair, my back freezes and I get stuck in the chair and cannot get out. Although my digestion has massively improved, I still have eventration on the right abdominal area near my hip where the surgeons had to cut me in half. I have a visible bulge in my right lower abdomen near my hip, which looks and acts like a hernia, but it's not a hernia yet. I was advised by the medical doctors referred as eventration. Often, I have to wear a torso compression wrap for support. I definitely have a lot of scars on my body, which make great war stories.

Once my back was stable, I underwent treatment and surgery for my cervical. The same team of surgeons at Cedar Sinai were involved. An x-ray and MRI scan revealed three disintegrated discs in my neck. My C3 was laying on C6, with bone spurs into my cranial and nasal areas. The surgeons entered through the front of my neck, had to jack up my cervical spine, and inserted cadaver bone, plates, cage, and screws. They kept me four days for observation and I was released. Of all the surgeries I've ever had, and I've had quite a few, this was the least painful and complicated. I think the worst thing I possibly did while recovering was to look up or turn my head.

Several years after these surgeries, my health improved immensely. Although I still underwent occasional injections or had spinal headaches, they were minimal compared to what I had before. Recently, I had trouble drinking or eating food for several days, and passed out as a result, striking my jaw against the bathroom counter and landing on the floor. I had to drive myself to the ER for treatment. My jaw was severely bruised, and I had a concussion. The ER MD determined my stomach had quit working, and I had a stomach blockage. I was admitted and tests were run. A large tube was inserted through my nose and down to my stomach. Two pints of undigested food and fluids were sucked out of my stomach. A feeding tube was inserted into my arm. The MDs at the hospital believed the medications I had been on for my orthopedic issues had caused a breakdown in my system. Eventually, they gave me an antibiotic to clear up an infection in my small intestine, and I was able to eat. The treating MD could not decide if my gall bladder needed to be removed. The MD decided not to remove the gallbladder, since it was healthy; however, it was sick from the infection. I was discharged after ten days. A day later, I was doubled over in pain, with abdominal pain that radiated into my back, similar to child labor cramps. I was taken back to the emergency room. The MD there believed my gallbladder didn't get better, and I had gotten sick because of my small intestine and stomach not working, so they did emergency gallbladder removal surgery. I was admitted for two more days.

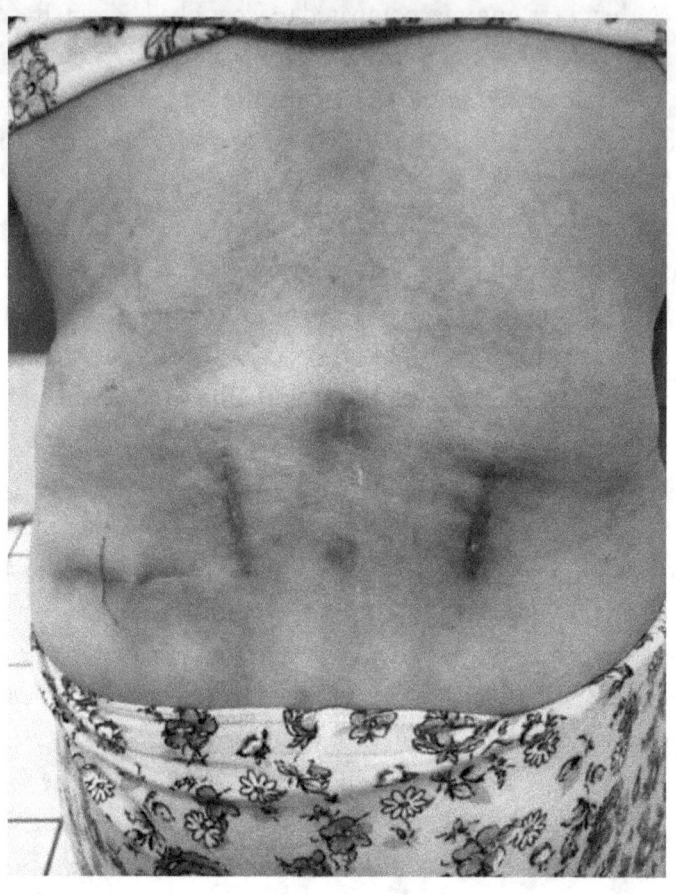

Here's a picture of my back a few years post-op after the removal of the implant. The doctor that I was referred to for orthopedic aftercare decided to remove plates and screws from my spine since my spine surgery had been successfully fused.

The removal of the plates and screws allowed for better movement and flexibility.

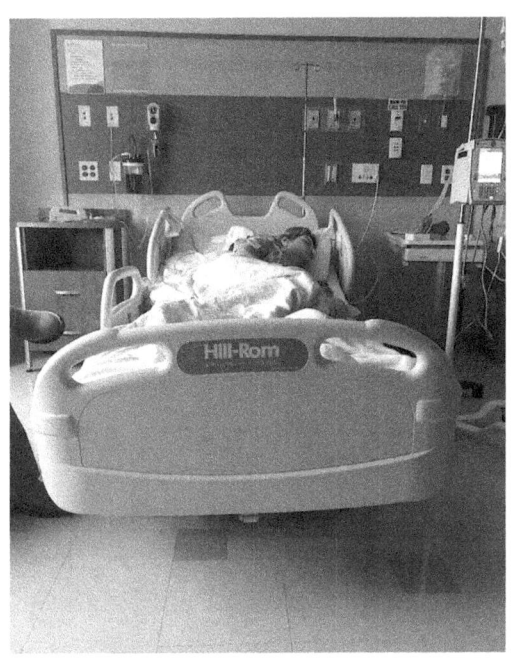
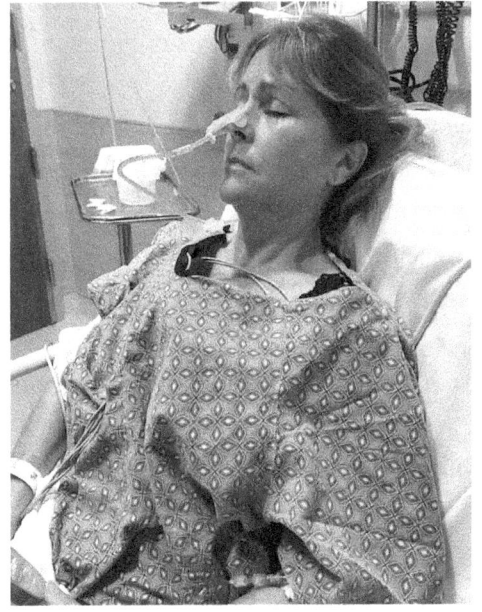

To this day, I still have random trouble with my digestion, back pain, neuropathy in my legs, mild headaches, and lymphedema. I learned that lymphedema is chronic, and never goes away. Although it may balance and go into submission, a simple paper cut, scratch, burn, or bruise causes the lymphedema to flare up. When this happens, my bladder won't empty on it's own, and requires me to use a self-catheter. Usually, the flare up dissipates after a few days to a week.

In conclusion, it is my hope that my experiences and story somehow reaches the right people in need of information or help. I don't want people to suffer like I did. I pray this story will lead you in the right direction to healing. Please be candid with your doctors and surgeons. Don't be afraid to ask questions. Blood allergy orthopedic implant tests can be done all over the United States. Simply research this online. If known allergies are present prior to surgery, please do research with the implant components. Discuss with your doctors and research the outcome reviews online. I am still recovering thirteen years later, but in a better place physically, mentally, and spiritually. Each person has different pains and tolerances. It is up to each person to seek within themselves for inner strength. We are all stronger than we think. The human body is quite amazing, but our minds are even more powerful. If anyone reading this thinks their medical issues are similar to what I had experienced, tell your doctor. Ask questions regarding getting proper care and treatment. Do your research like I did. Don't be afraid to get counseling for any mental health resulting from medical issues. I wish all the best to my readers and send love and light your way. God bless.

www.ingramcontent.com/pod-product-compliance
Lightning Source LLC
LaVergne TN
LVHW021744060526
838200LV00052B/3466